Look at a mirror and open your mouth. What do you see?

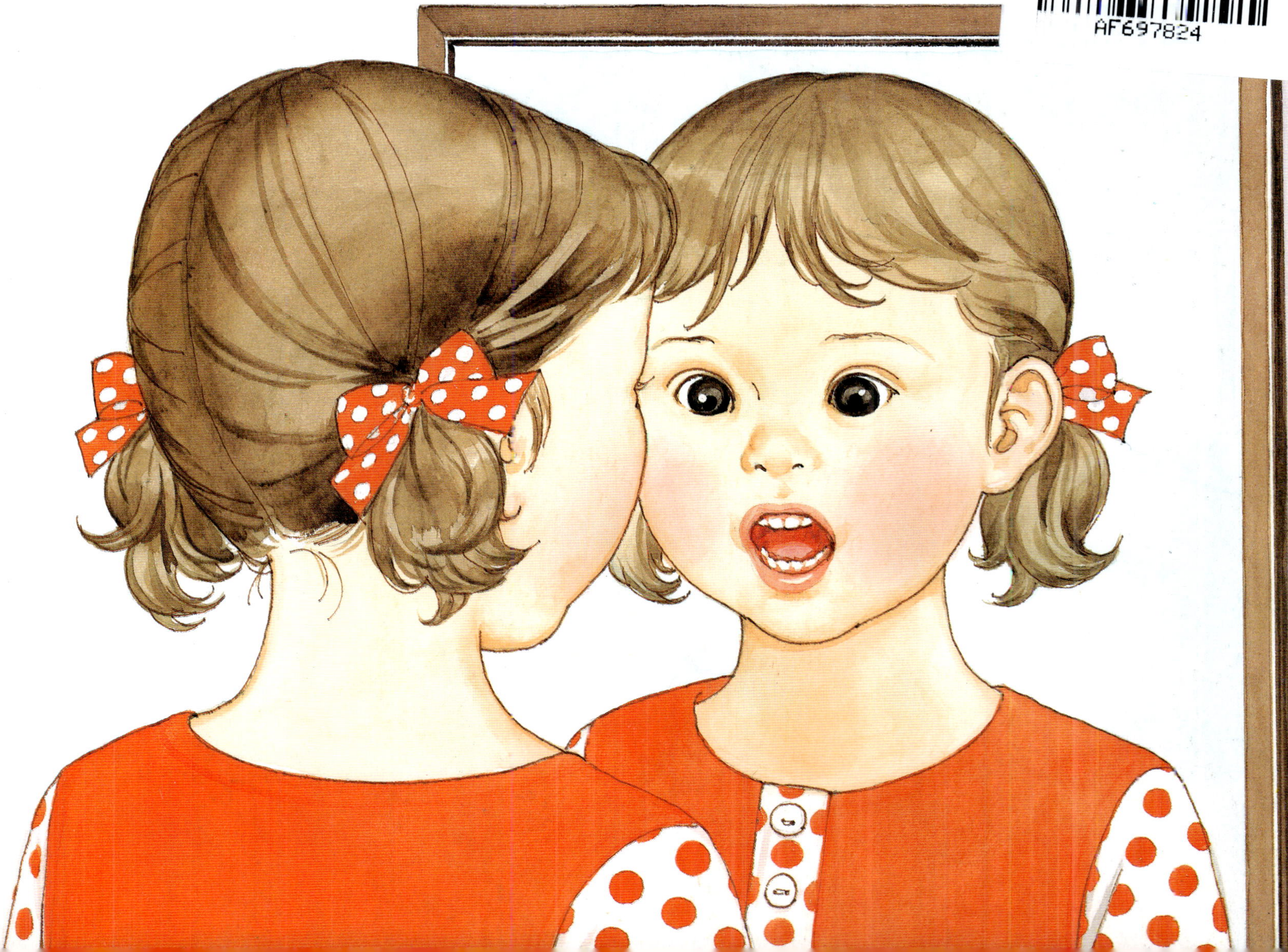

This is what the inside of your mouth looks like.

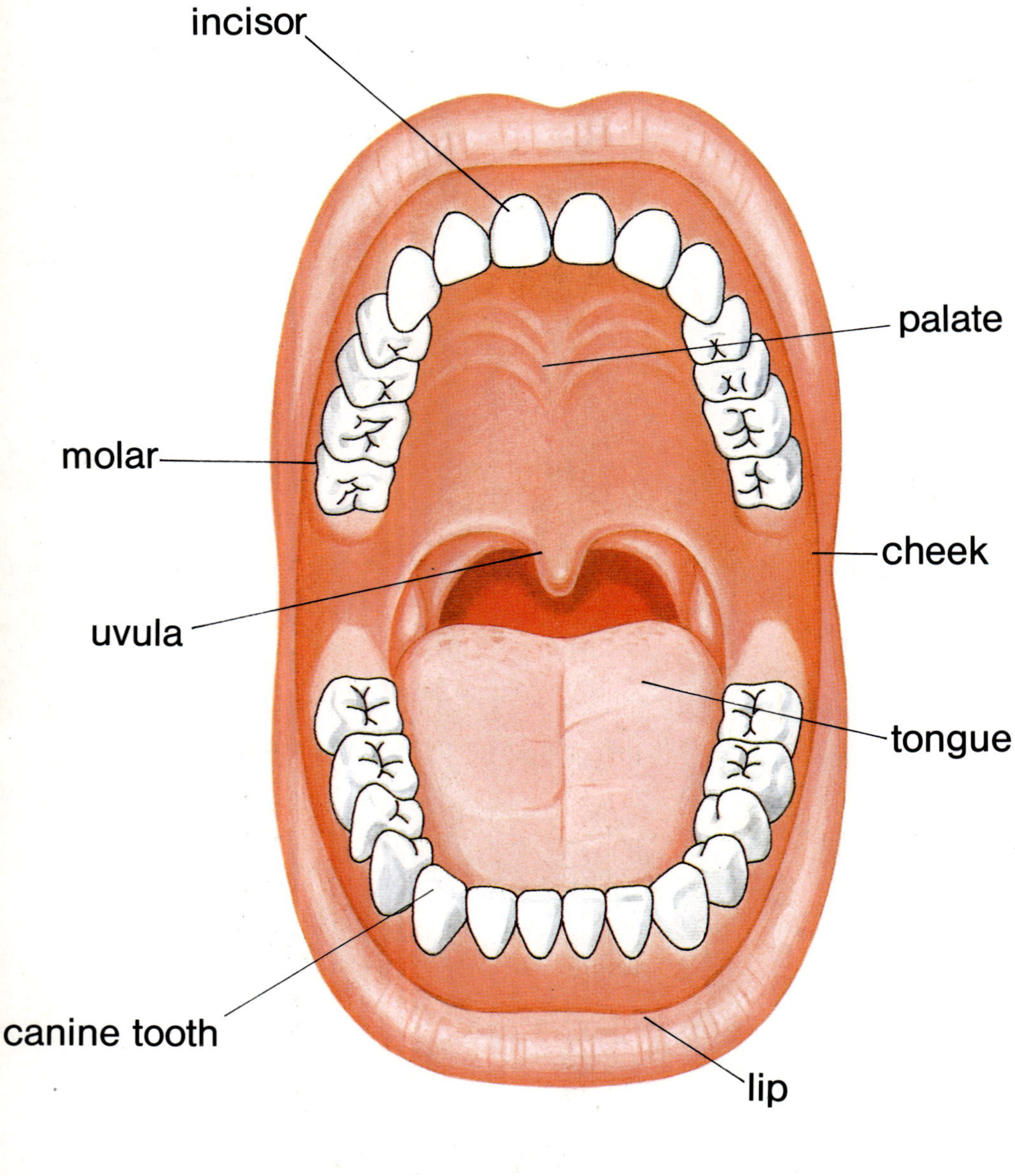

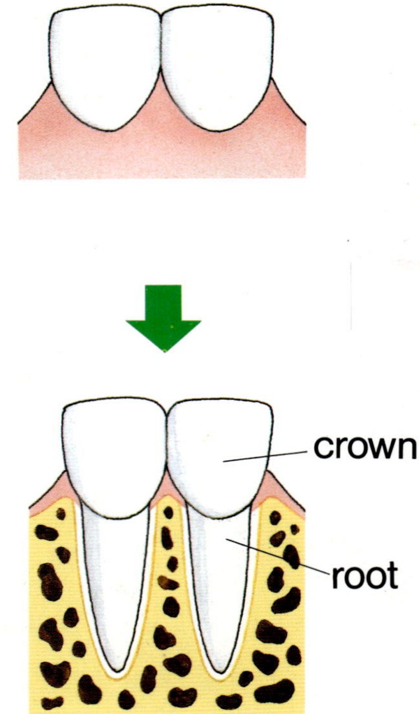

Each tooth has two parts — a crown (the part you see) and one or more roots attaching it to the jaw.

Are any of your teeth loose?

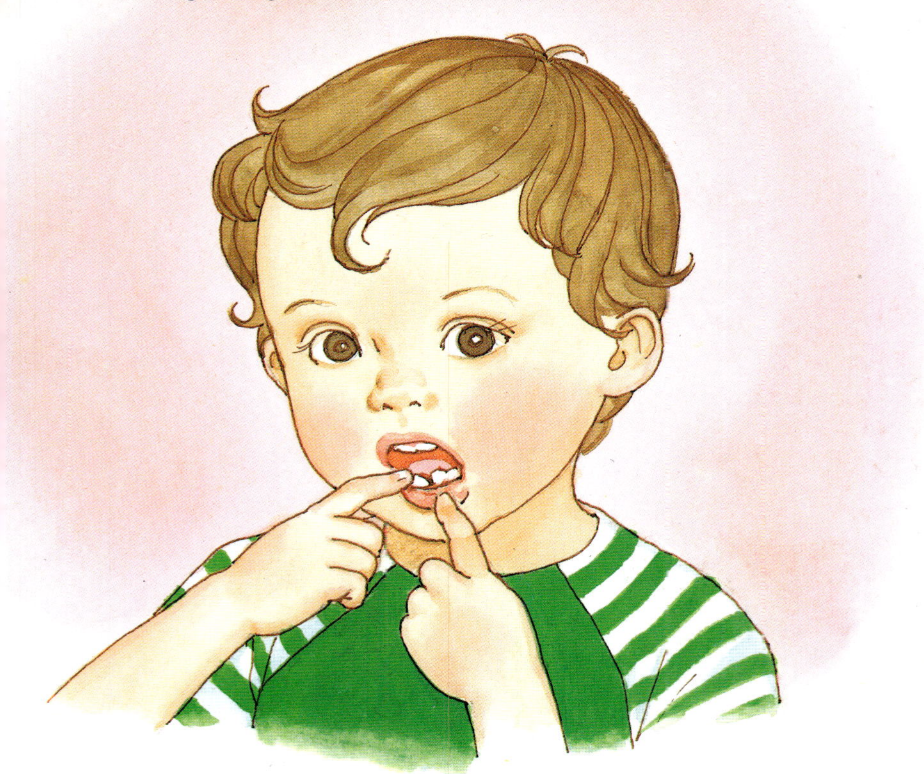

Teeth that become loose are baby teeth.

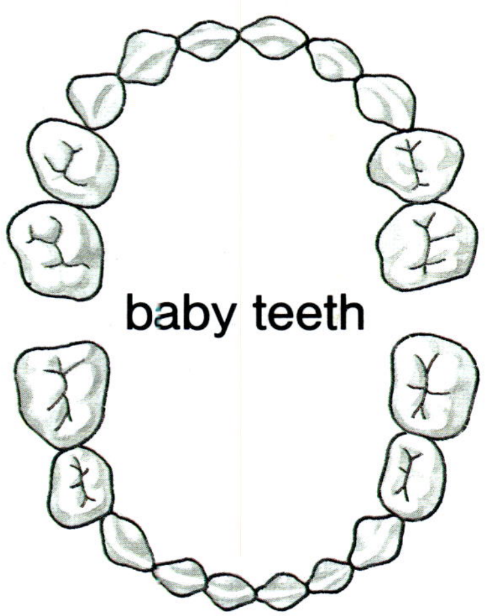

Baby teeth come in when we are very small. When we are six or so, we begin to lose them, and our permanent teeth appear.

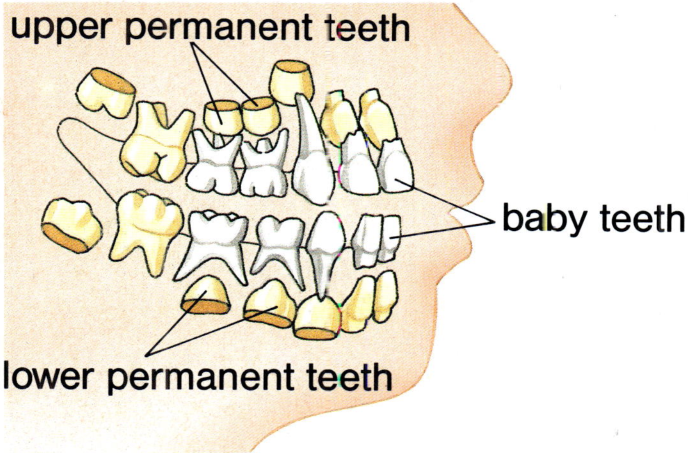

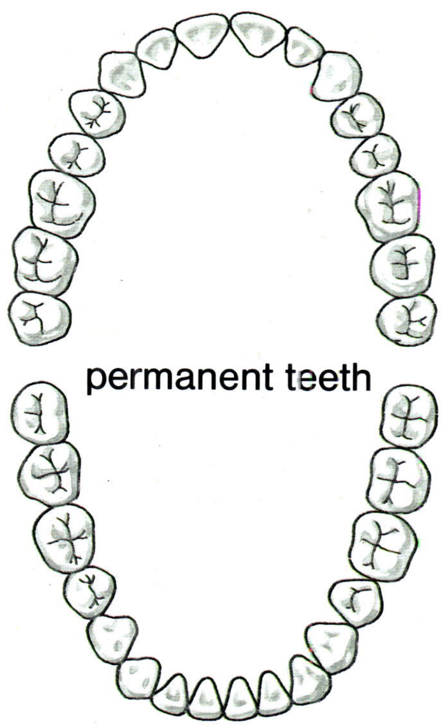

Why do we have teeth?

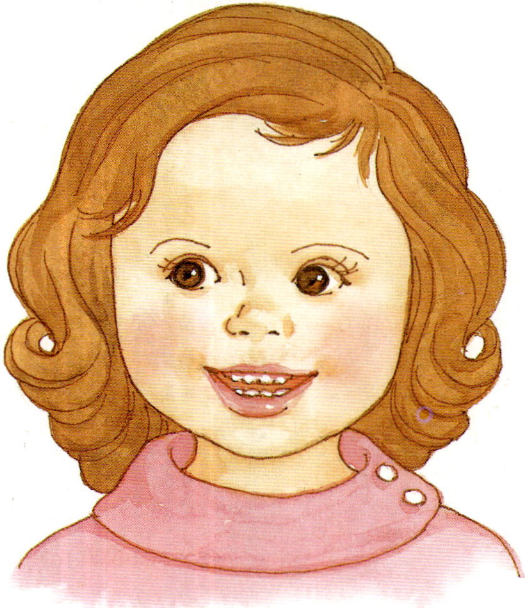

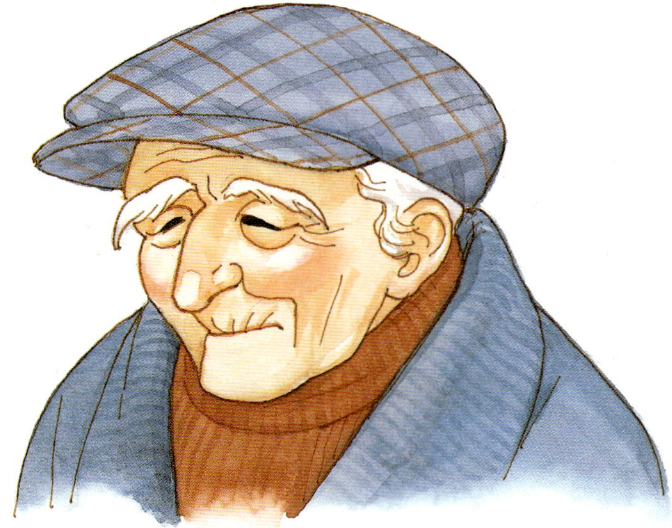

Teeth are a part of your face. Without teeth, you would seem different. Nice white teeth look best.

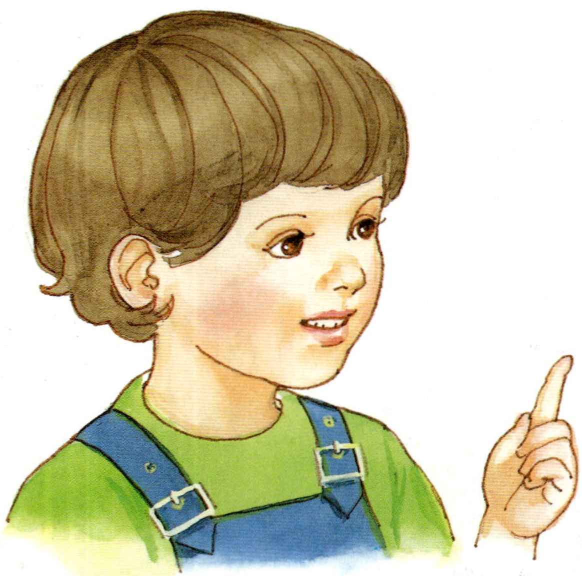

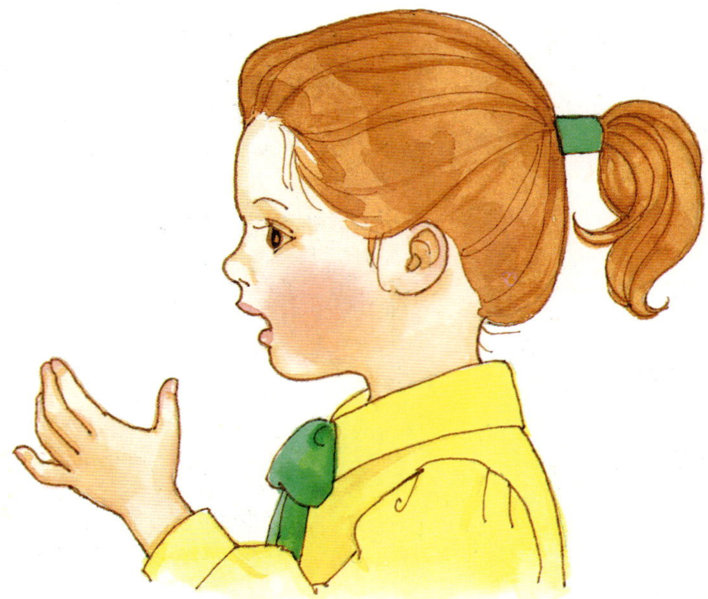

Teeth help us pronounce words. Without teeth, it is harder to talk.

But the most important work our teeth do is chewing our food.

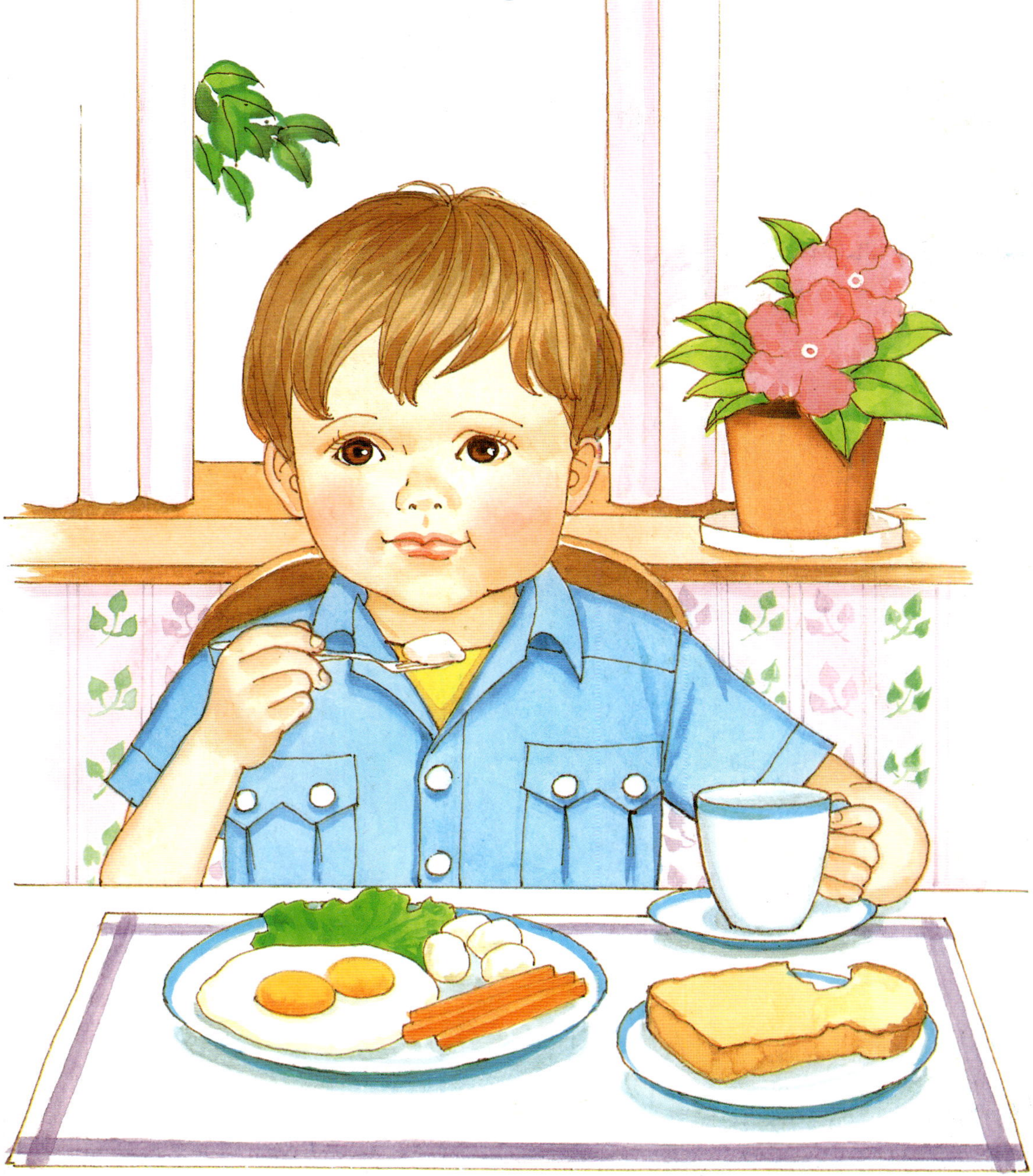

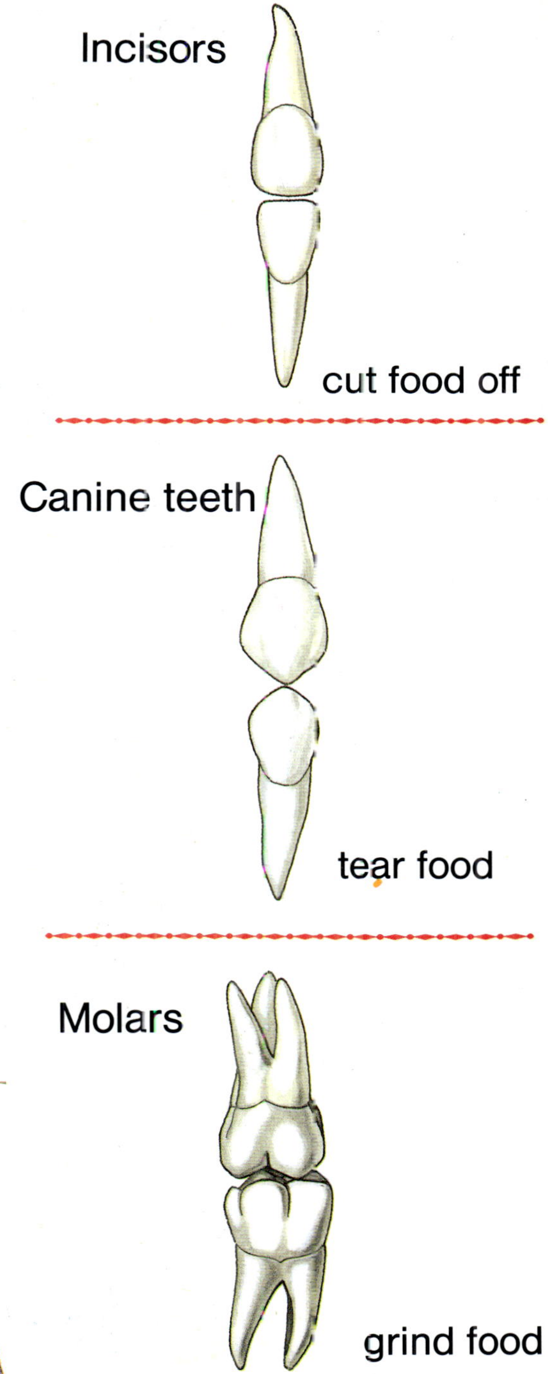

When we eat, our teeth are helped by a digestive juice in our mouths. It is called saliva. It moistens and softens our food. When we think of something good, our mouths water and produce more saliva.

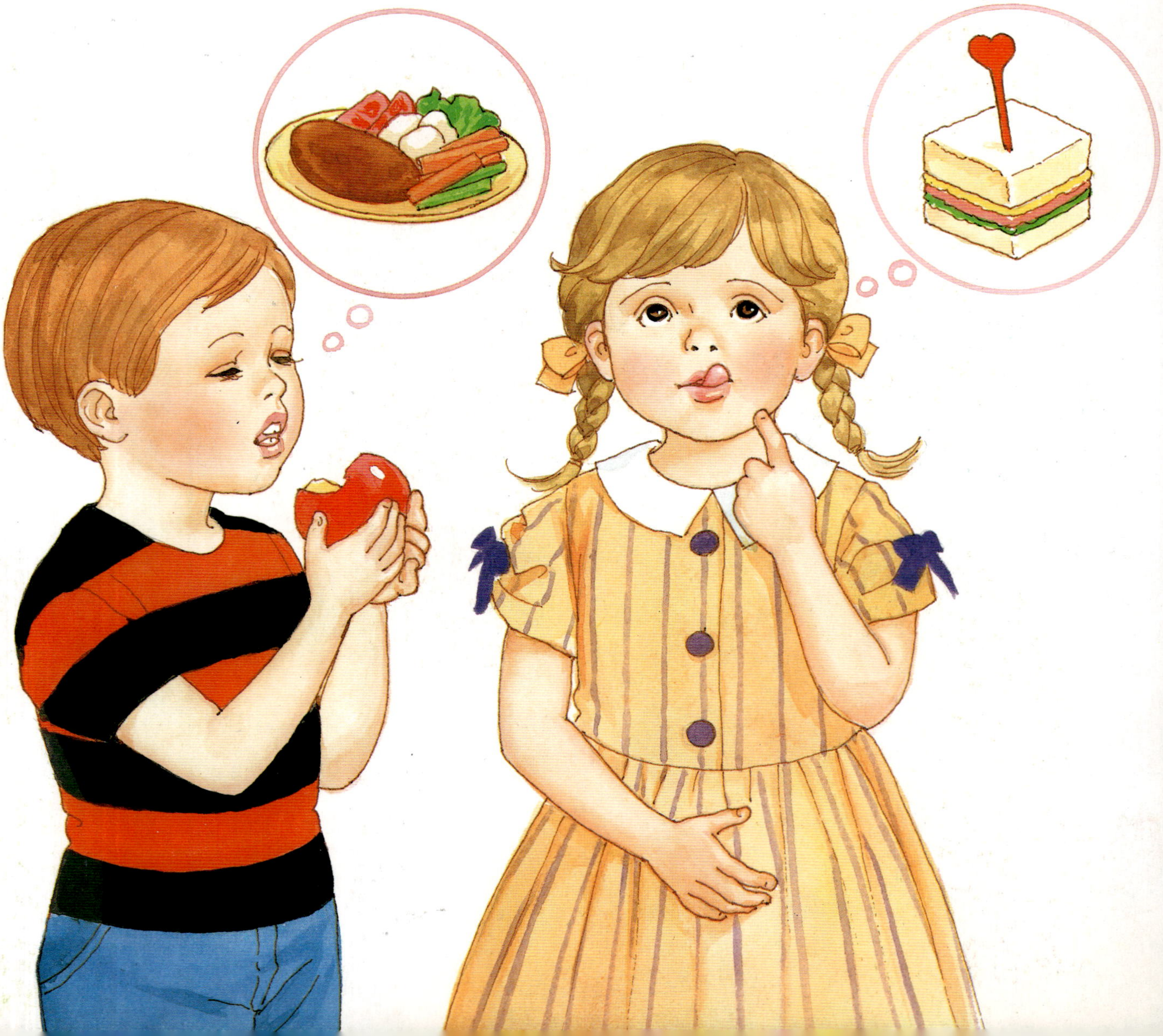

We taste things with our tongues. Look closely at the surface of your tongue. It is covered with small bumps. These are taste buds. There are four kinds, one for each basic kind of taste.

Sour

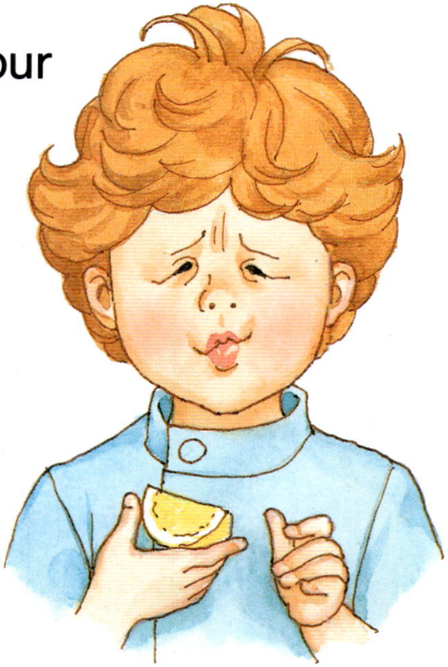

Bitter

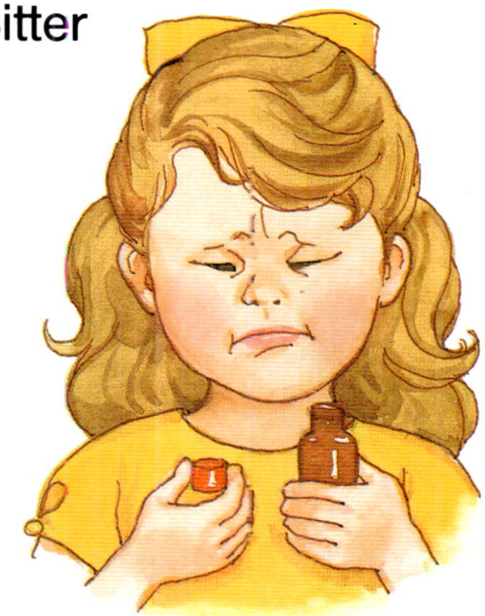

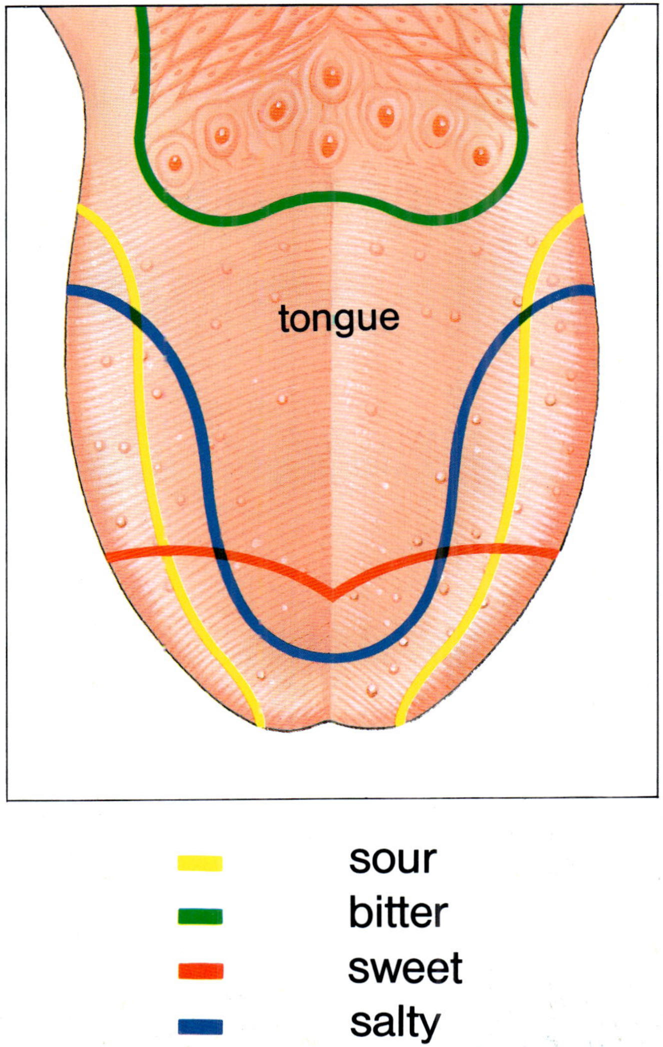

Sweet

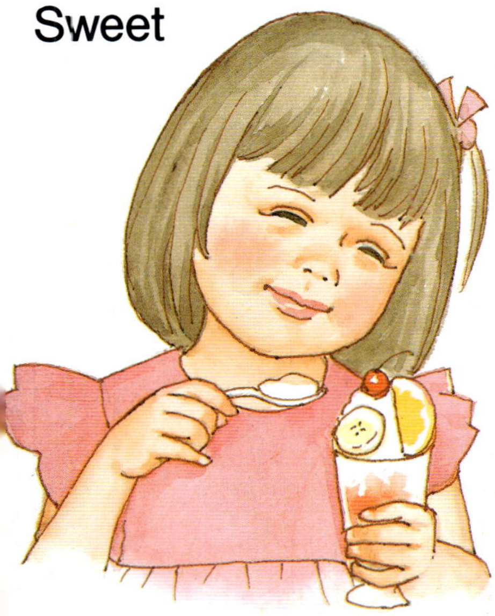

Salty

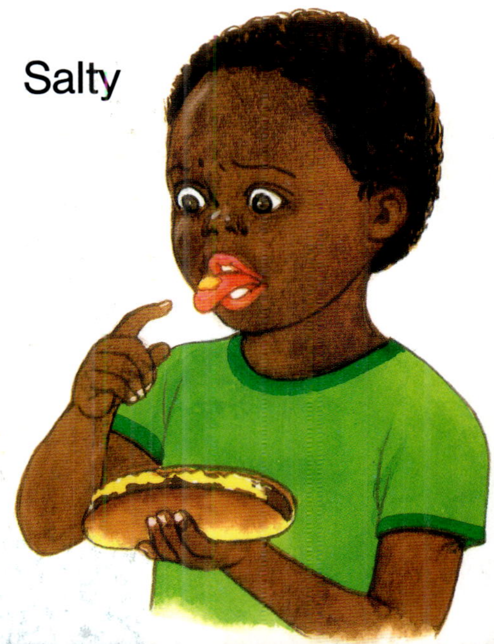

What kinds of food do you like?

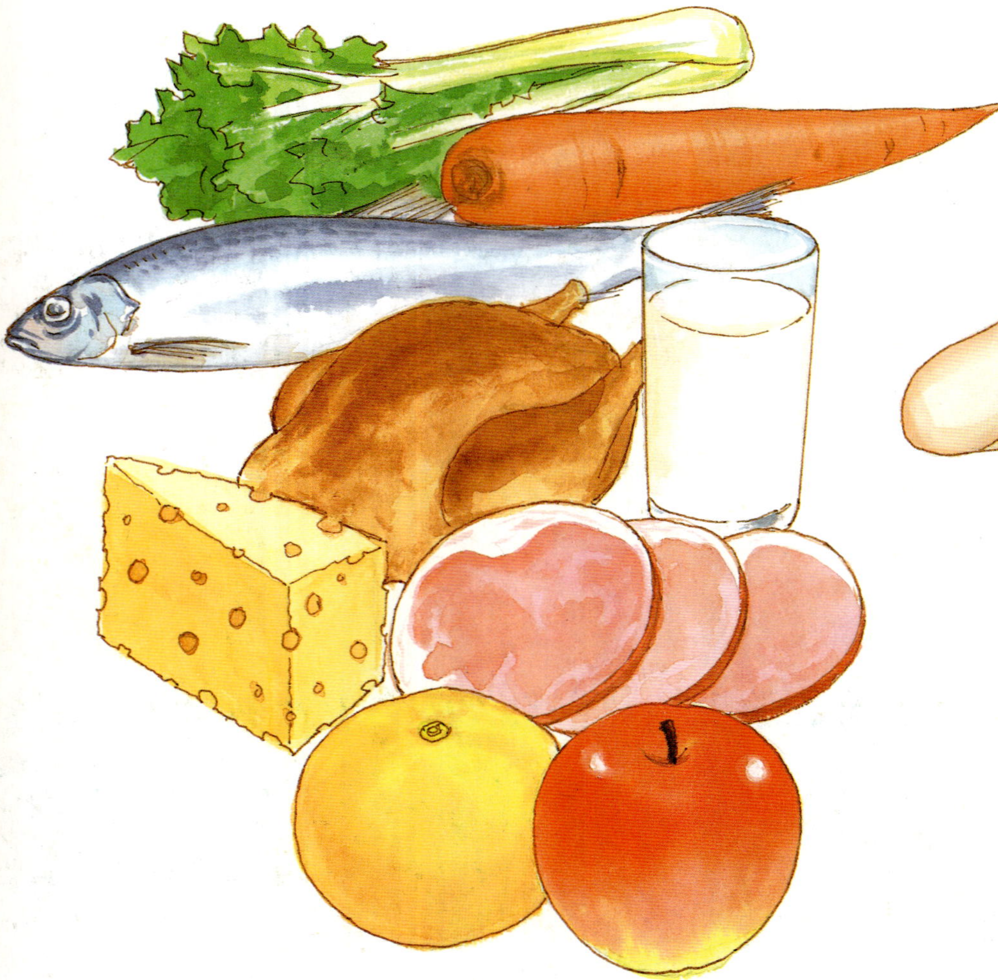

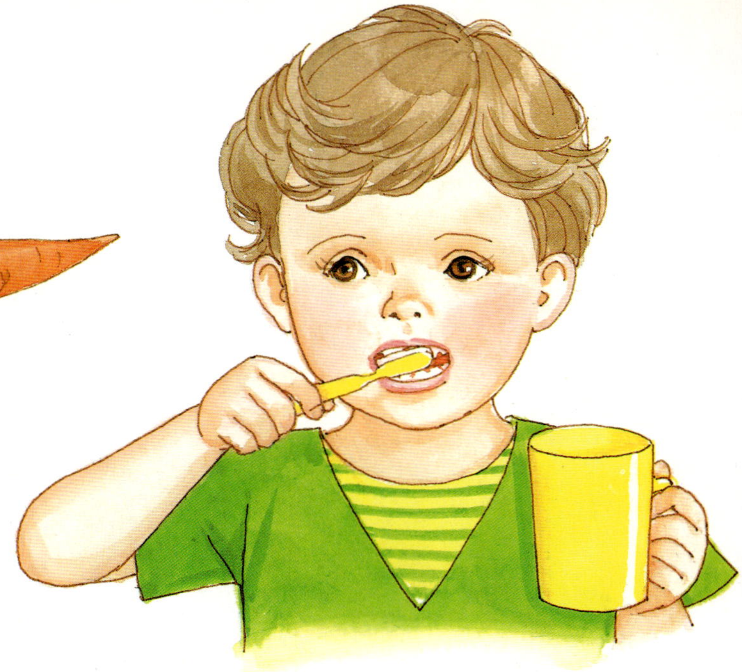

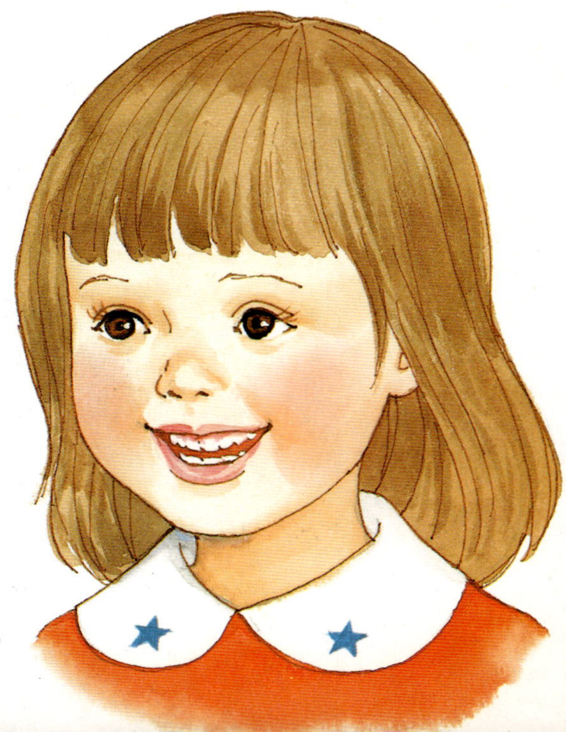

Foods with quality proteins, vitamins A, C, and D, calcium, and phosphorus are good for your teeth. Brush your teeth after eating. Keep your teeth healthy.

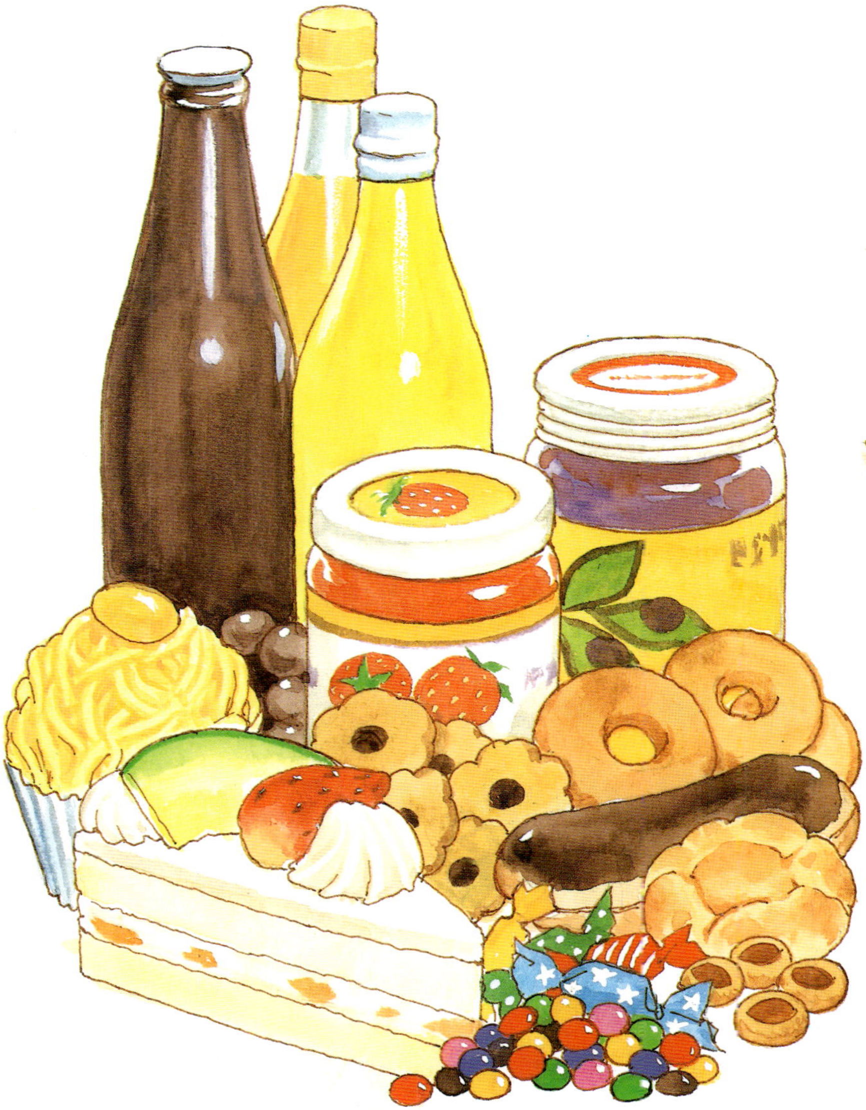

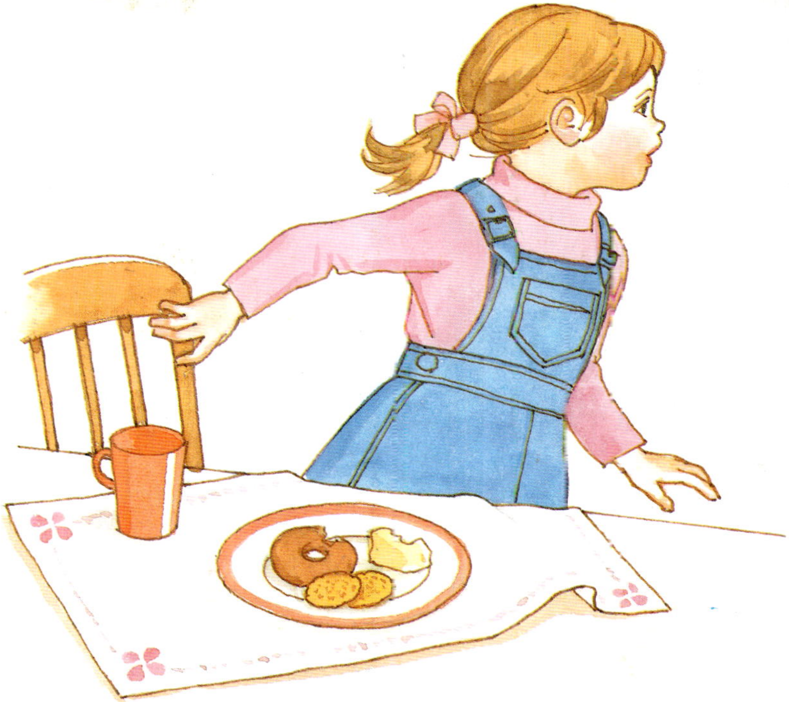

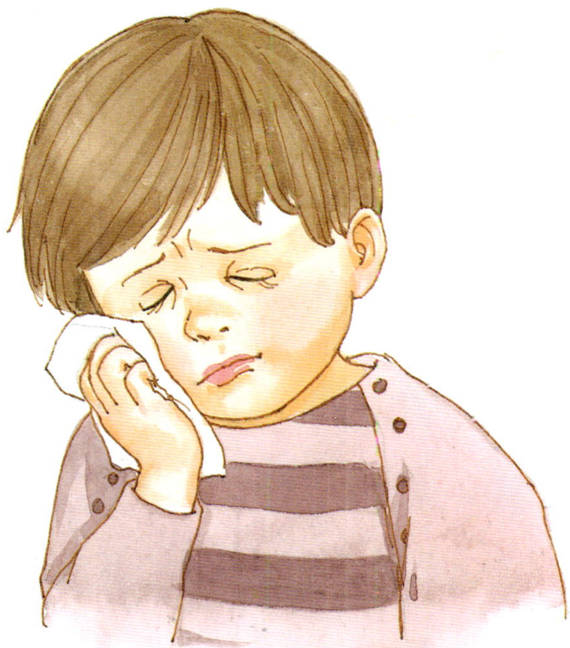

Sweet, sticky foods cause cavities. If you eat them and do not brush your teeth, you will have trouble with decay.

This is how teeth decay.

Food particles gather on your teeth and combine with bacteria to form a substance called plaque. Then, acids are produced. They attack your teeth and destroy the enamel, causing cavities. At first, there is little or no pain. But the cavities are growing, all the same.

The structure of the tooth

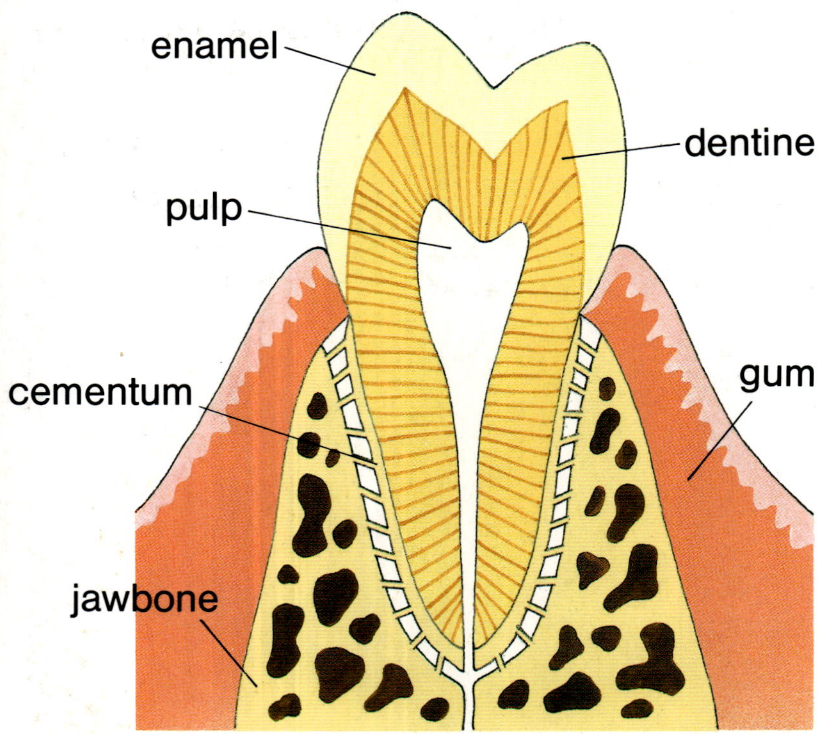

Growth of a cavity

The enamel is broken down.
(At first, there is not much pain.)

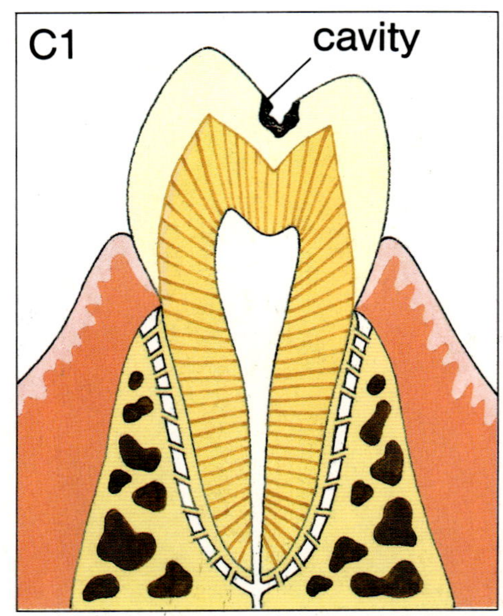

Can you find any cavities in these spots?

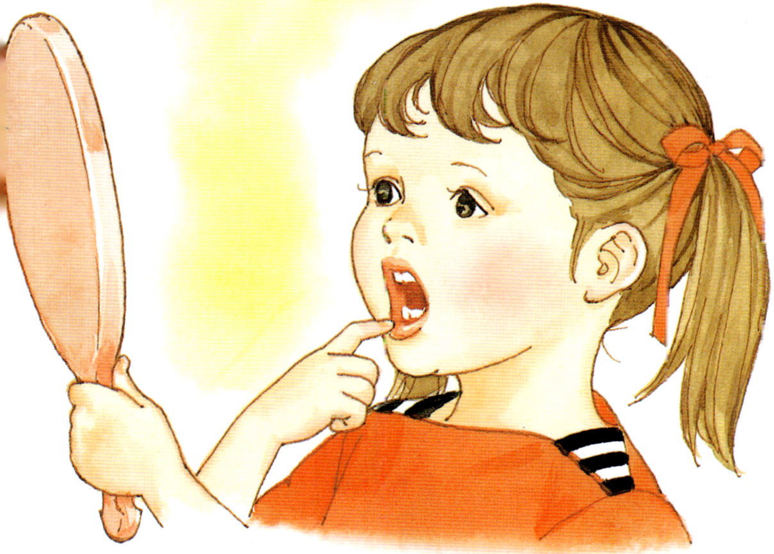

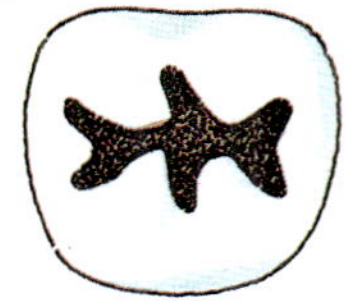

The top surfaces of teeth

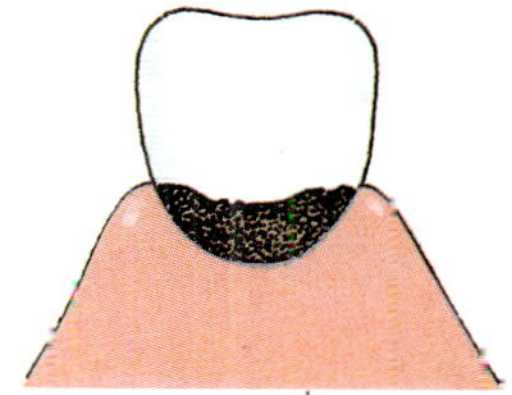

The edges of teeth and gums

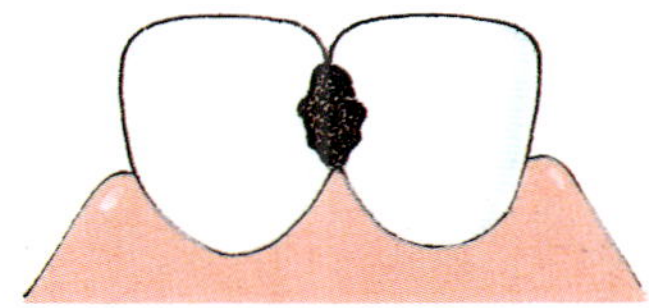

The space between teeth

Decay spreads to the dentine.
(Teeth grow sensitive to water.)

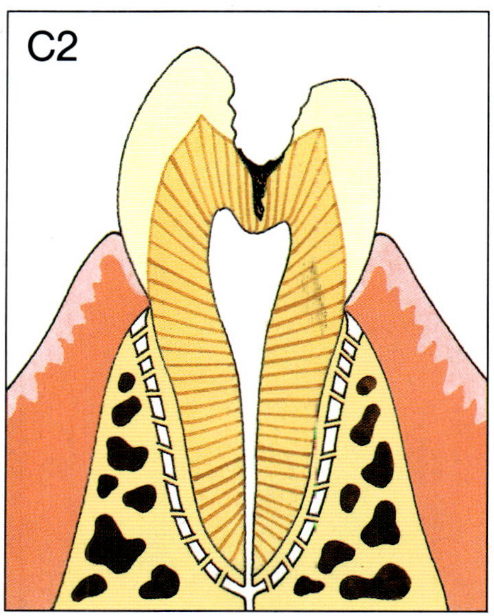

The pulp layer is attacked.
(You have a toothache.)

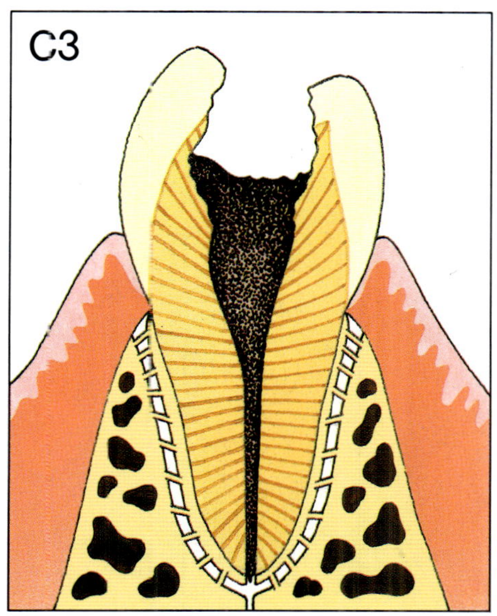

The crown is destroyed.
(Only roots remain.)

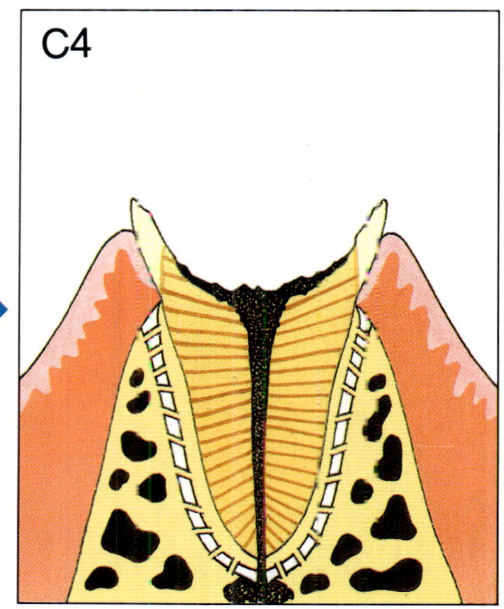

To have strong teeth, we must take care of them.

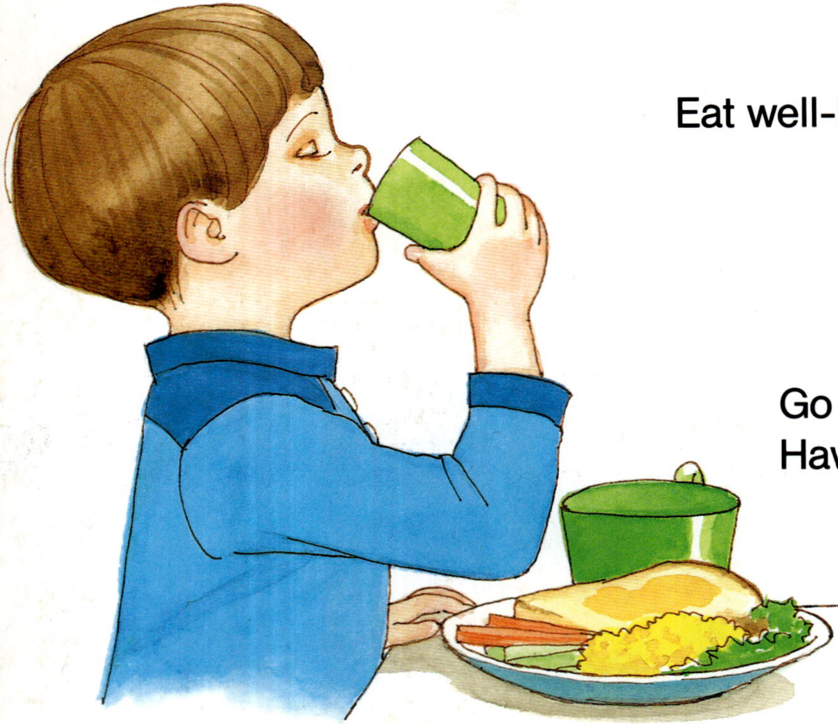

Eat well-balanced meals at regular meal-times.

Go to the dentist for regular examinations.
Have cavities treated early.

Rinse your mouth and brush your teeth, especially after eating.

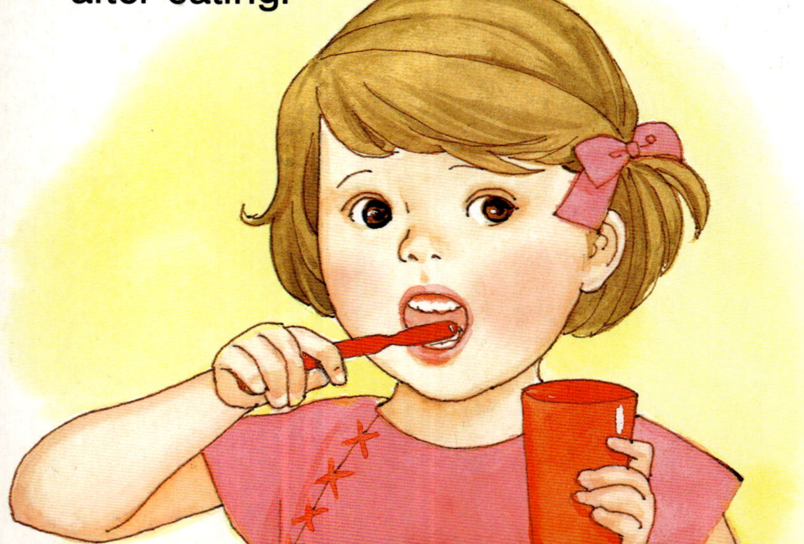

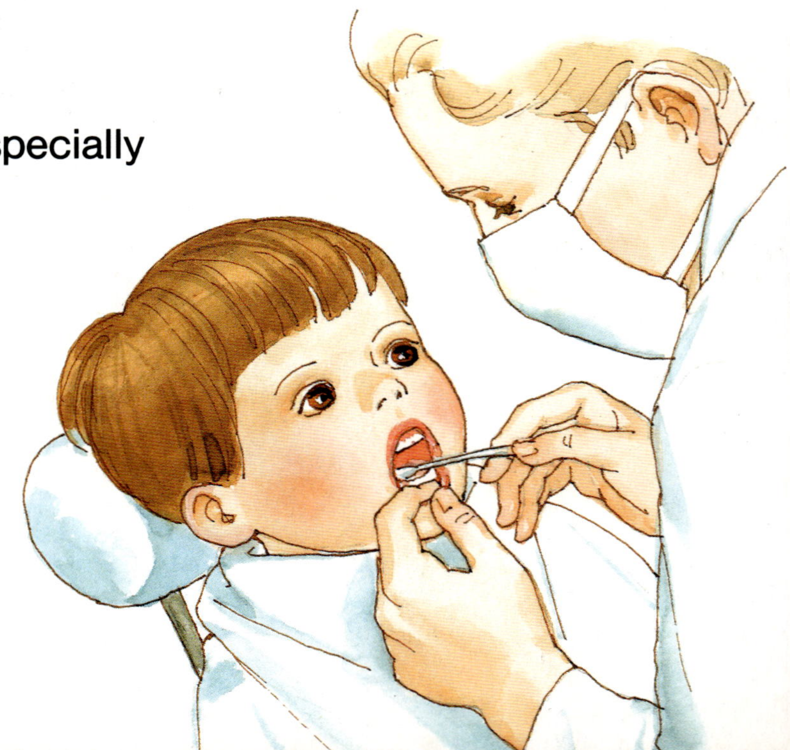